Hend RIAHI

Radio-clinical correlation in degenerative narrow lumbar canal

Hend RIAHI

Radio-clinical correlation in degenerative narrow lumbar canal

ScienciaScripts

Imprint

Any brand names and product names mentioned in this book are subject to trademark, brand or patent protection and are trademarks or registered trademarks of their respective holders. The use of brand names, product names, common names, trade names, product descriptions etc. even without a particular marking in this work is in no way to be construed to mean that such names may be regarded as unrestricted in respect of trademark and brand protection legislation and could thus be used by anyone.

Cover image: www.ingimage.com

This book is a translation from the original published under ISBN 978-620-6-71080-6.

Publisher:
Sciencia Scripts
is a trademark of
Dodo Books Indian Ocean Ltd. and OmniScriptum S.R.L publishing group

120 High Road, East Finchley, London, N2 9ED, United Kingdom
Str. Armeneasca 28/1, office 1, Chisinau MD-2012, Republic of Moldova, Europe
Printed at: see last page
ISBN: 978-620-7-61478-3

TABLE OF CONTENTS

INTRODUCTION

Degenerative narrow lumbar canal is a frequent anatomical and clinical entity [1,2]. It is defined anatomically by a reduction in the diameter of the medullary canal due to arthrosic phenomena, resulting in compression of the nerve and vascular structures it contains, and clinically by a painful spinal syndrome and a radicular syndrome mainly affecting the roots from L3 to S1 [1,2]. Thanks to advances in imaging and the ageing of the population, there has been an increase in the frequency of diagnosis [3,4].

The course of this condition can be serious, with sensory-motor and genital-sphincter complications [5,6].

The causes of radicular pain are not unequivocal. They probably comprise several components: anatomical, neuropathic, vascular and biochemical [1,3,7]. This pathophysiological complexity could probably explain the variety of symptoms and, in part, the lack of anatomical-clinical parallelism [4].

Specialists have been able to establish a definition of lumbar canal stenosis, which must have an anteroposterior diameter of less than 10mm [8]. Some also consider the surface area of the dural sac, in axial section on imaging, to make the diagnosis of lumbar canal stenosis. An area of less than 100mm2 represents relative narrowness, whereas an area of less than 75mm2 represents absolute stenosis [8,9]. These two radiological parameters have a limitation: multiple studies have shown that there is no relationship between the size of the dural sac and the symptoms reported by the patient [10-18].

The gold standard is spinal cord MRI, which provides a precise morphological illustration [4,19-21]. It studies the degree of stenosis of the rootlets in the dural sac, defining the Schizas classification [8,22].

Could there be an association between this classification and clinical symptoms? The aim of our work was to study the correlation between the Schizas classification and clinical manifestations of degenerative narrow lumbar canal.

I. TYPE OF STUDY

This was a descriptive, evaluative and retrospective study, carried out in the La Rabta orthopaedic department and focusing on patients with a degenerative narrow lumbar canal.

II. CHOICE OF SAMPLE

We collated 82 patient files identified from the archive notebooks (patients followed and/or hospitalised in the department, whether operated on or not, between January 2010 and December 2021) with the coding keyword: narrow lumbar canal.

II. 1. Inclusion criteria :

In our study, we included patients :

- Who had a degenerative narrow lumbar canal.

- Which were examined before surgery.

- Having an MRI of the lumbar spine.

- Off medication for more than 15 days and off rehabilitation for more than 45 days.
- No vascular claudication on examination.

II. 2. Non-inclusion criteria :

This work does not include :

- Files not containing MRI images and reports.

- Narrow lumbar spinal canal of traumatic, tumoral, iatrogenic or infectious origin.

II. 3. Exclusion criteria :

We have excluded :

- Files with incomplete data.

- Cases with poor quality MRI images and incomplete reports which prevent us from properly determining the Schizas classification.
- Patients with a chronic inflammatory rheumatic disease that may affect the spine.
- Patients with a sensory-motor deficit linked to a paralysing neurological disease.

III. METHODS

Data collection :

Our working method consisted of collecting epidemiological, anamnestic, clinical and radiological data, using a data processing form (**Appendix 1**), which were then reported in an Excel table. We carried out a descriptive and statistical study, analysing the data using SPSS software.

We collected the following data for each of our patients:

II. 1 Epidemiological data :

- Age.

- Genre.

- Medical and surgical history.

II.2 Data from the examination :

The main complaints that emerged from the history were :

- Low back pain: its onset, intensity, impact on daily activities and response to medical treatment.

- A patient's permanent functional disability using the Oswestry disability index (**Appendix 2**): This was designed to give us information on how spinal pathology has affected the ability to cope in everyday life. It involved answering all sections of the questionnaire. The final result was expressed as a percentage of disability [23].

- Pain intensity using the visual analogue scale [24-26] (**Appendix**

3).

- Intermittent neurogenic claudication, which was only relieved by bending forward or sitting down. This was explained by the fact that flexion of the spine increases the diameter of the lumbar canal and vice versa for extension [1,3,27]. Vascular claudication was the differential diagnosis, which could be ruled out by a good history and careful clinical examination [28] (**Appendix 4**).

- Limitation of walking perimeter. To facilitate the work, we divided the cohort into three groups in an arbitrary manner in the absence of a clear consensus.

Group 1 with a walking perimeter >500m.

Group 2 with a reduced walking perimeter of between 100 and 500m.

Group 3 with a very reduced walking perimeter <100m.

- Radiculalgia: location, time to onset, uni- or bilateral, uni- or multi-radicular.

- -Genito-sphincter disorders.

II. 3 Clinical examination :

A physical examination focusing on the musculoskeletal and neurological systems was carried out:

- A postural syndrome: accentuation or reduction of one of the spinal curves, the presence of a scoliotic attitude, looking for compensation for a sagittal imbalance of the spine by flexing the hip or knees.

- A spinal syndrome: pain, contractures of the paravertebral muscles, stiffness of the spine by measuring the distance between the fingers and the ground and the Schober index [29,30].

- A radicular syndrome: by the Sonnette sign and the manoeuvres of

Lasègue [31].

- Whether or not there is a sensory and/or motor deficit by muscle

testing [32,33] (**Appendix 5)**, cauda equina syndrome or pyramidal

syndrome.

- Appreciate muscle tone.

- Research into osteotendinous reflexes.

II. 4 Imaging data :

The lumbar spinal canal is made up of two zones, a central zone and a

lateral zone, which may be constitutionally stenotic or acquired,

resulting in compression of the vascular and neural elements once they

reach a certain degree of narrowness [3,34]. Imaging assesses the

elements involved, the degree of stenosis, its topography and any

dynamic component.

Constitutional stenosis is most often seen at the time of the onset of a

secondary degenerative factor [2,35].

The degenerative anomalies that can combine to narrow the lumbar

canal are as follows [19,36]:

- Degenerative disc disease with herniated disc.

- Discarthrosis with corporal osteophytosis.

- Osteoarthritis of the zygapophysis, sometimes associated with a

synovial cyst.

- Thickened, calcified and ossified ligaments (yellow ligament, posterior common vertebral ligament).

- Hyperostosis of the blades.

Axial-section T2-sequence MRI images of the lumbar canal were taken of our patients. We assessed the ratio between the area occupied by the rootlets of the cauda equina and the area occupied by the cerebrospinal fluid. This morphological description defines the Schizas classification [8,22], which is composed of four grades: A1-4, B, C and D in ascending order of stenosis severity (**Figure 1**).

Grade A: no stenosis or minor stenosis
A1: dorsally arranged rootlets occupying less than half the surface area of the dural sac.

A2: rootlets arranged dorsally in a horseshoe shape.
A3: dorsally arranged rootlets occupying more than half the surface area of the dural sac.

A4: centrally located rootlets occupying most of the surface area of the dural sac.

Grade B: moderate stenosis: the rootlets occupy the entire dural sac, but the rootlets can still be individualised.

Grade C: severe stenosis: no recognisable rootlets with complete effacement of the cerebrospinal fluid space, but epidural fat is present posteriorly.

Grade D: extreme stenosis: no recognisable rootlets and no epidural fat behind.

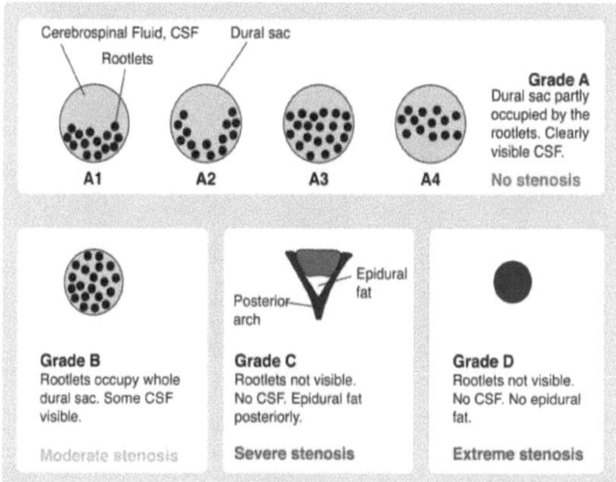

Figure 1: Morphological classification of grades of lumbar canal stenosis [8].

Figures 2 to 5 show axial-section T2 MRI images of the lumbar spine:

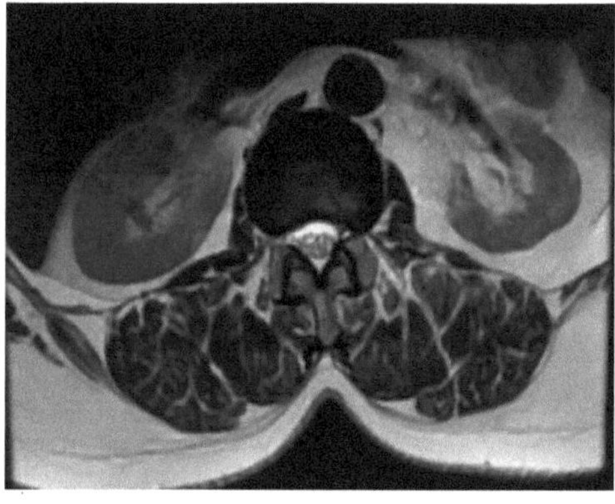

Figure 2: Axial section of a T2 sequence MRI scan of the lumbar spine showing minor stenosis with rootlets occupying more than half the dural sac (Schizas stage A3).

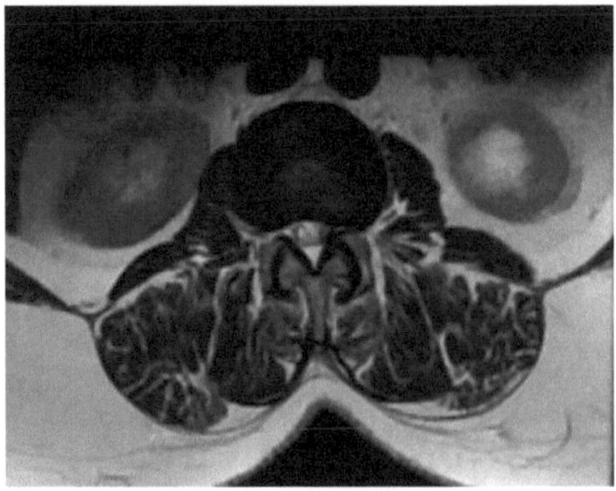

Figure 3: Axial section of a T2 sequence MRI scan of the lumbar spine showing moderate stenosis with the appearance of rootlets occupying the entire dural sac, but the rootlets can still be individualised (Schizas stage B).

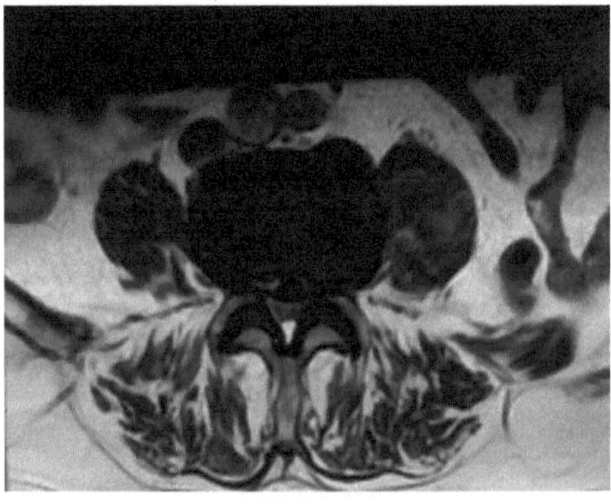

Figure 4: Axial section of a T2 sequence MRI scan of the lumbar spine showing severe stenosis with unrecognisable rootlets and complete effacement of the CSF space, but epidural fat is present posteriorly (Schizas Stage C).

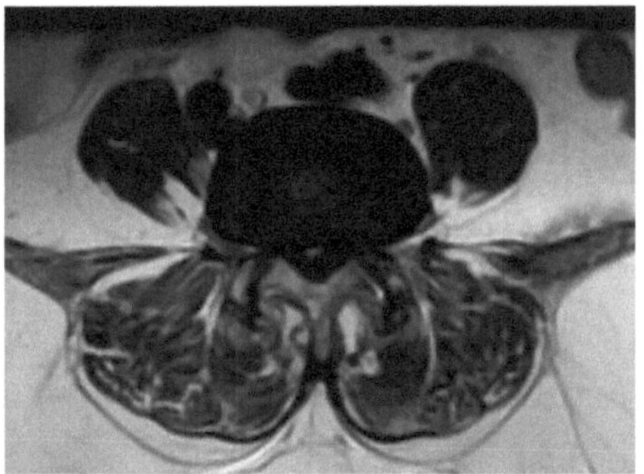

Figure 5: Axial section of a T2 sequence MRI scan of the lumbar spine showing extreme stenosis with unrecognisable rootlets and no epidural fat behind (Schizas Grade D).

IV. ETHICAL CONSIDERATIONS AND CONFLICTS OF INTEREST

We declare that there are no conflicts of interest in relation to this work. We also guarantee the confidentiality of the data collected and have implemented security measures for sending, receiving and storing this data.

V. BIBLIOGRAPHIC RESEARCH

The keywords used in the literature search were: narrow lumbar canal, MRI, clinical, signs and symptoms, classification, correlation.

Search engines consulted :

- PubMed

- ScienceDirect

- EM Consult

- Springler

I. DESCRIPTIVE STUDY

I.1 Age and gender :

The average age of the cases was 58, with extremes of 39 and 80.There was a predominance of women, with 47 women (57%) and 35 men (43%), with a sex ratio of 0.74. The age distribution is shown in the diagram below **(Figure 6)**.

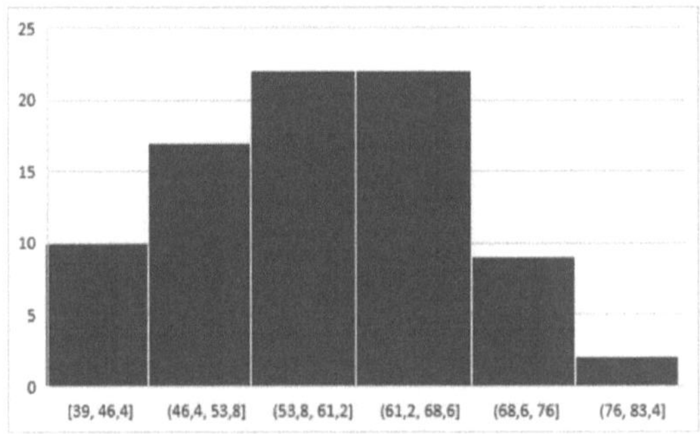

Figure 6: Age distribution of cases.

I.2 Development time :

The time between the onset of symptoms and the first consultation varies from 1 year to 12 years with an average of 04 years. The distribution of patients according to is shown in the diagram below **(Figure 7)**.

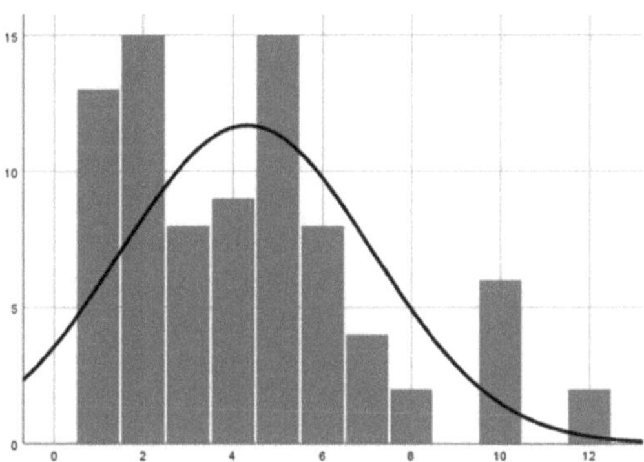

Figure 7: Distribution of patients according to duration of evolution.

I.3 Chronic low back pain :

Chronic low back pain was present in 96% of cases, whereas it was absent in in 4% of patients.

I.4 Radiculalgia :

All our patients suffered from radiculalgia. Radiculalgia was unilateral in 35 cases and bilateral in 47 cases. They were uniradicular in 77 cases, pluriradicular in 05 cases and poorly systematised in 11 cases. The topographical study of the roots showed a predominant involvement of the L5 root (38 cases) according to the following diagram **(figure 8)**.

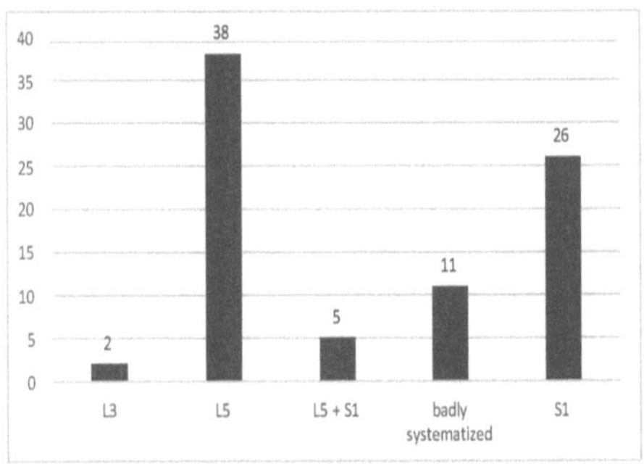

Figure 8: Distribution of patients according to type of radiculalgia

I.5 Intensity of pain :

Pain intensity was assessed using the VAS score. The average score was 7, with extremes of 4 and 9. The distribution of patients according to pain intensity using the VAS score is as follows shown in **Table I.**

Table I: Distribution of patients according to pain intensity.

	Workforce	Percentage
Mild pain [VAS 1-3]	0	0%
Moderate pain [VAS4-5]	23	28%
Severe pain [VAS6-7]	31	38%
Unbearable pain[EVA 8-10]	28	34%

I.6 Neurogenic claudication and gait perimeter :

Neurogenic claudication was found in 100% of patients. 30% of patients had a severe reduction in gait perimeter. The distribution of patients according to reduction in gait perimeter is shown in **Table II.**

Table II: Distribution of patients according to reduction in walking perimeter.

Walking perimeter	Workforce	Percentage
PM < 100m	25	30%
100m < PM < 500m	30	37%
PM > 500m	27	33%
Total	82	100%

The most frequent reason for stopping walking was neurogenic claudication, with a rate of 80%. The rest of the reasons were divided between recurrence of low back pain and pure low back pain. Thirty-two patients (32%) reported that hyperflexion or bending forward relieved their pain, while the others were forced to sit up.

I.7 Vesico-sphincter disorder :

In our series, 09 cases of urinary leakage, 12 cases of urinary urgency and 04 cases of sexual impotence were reported.

I.8 Functional capacity :

It was assessed by the Oswestry disability index (ODI). The mean score was 47%, with a minimum of 10% and a maximum of 90%.The breakdown of patients according to functional impairment is shown below in **table III**.

Table III: Distribution of patients according to functional impairment.

ODI score [%]	Workforce	Percentage
Minimal disability (0-20)	9	11%
Moderate disability (21-40)	27	33%
Severe disability (41-60)	26	32%
Cripple, pain impinges on all aspects of patient's life (61-80)	12	14%
Patients are bed-bound or exaggerating their symptoms (81-100)	8	10%
Total	82	100%

I.9 Clinical examination :

Spinal syndrome and postural syndrome:

- Spinal stiffness was found in 48 cases.

- Hyperlordosis in 05 cases.

- Loss of lumbar lordosis in 07 cases.

- Walking in a kyphosis or supermarket trolley position was noted in 03 cases.

- Scoliotic spinal deviation in 08 cases.

Radicular syndrome :

- Positive Lasègue sign (<40°) in 44 cases.

- Positive bell sign in 45 cases.

- Walking on the heel was impossible in 26 cases.

- Walking on tiptoes was impossible in 19 cases.

Sensory-motor deficit :

The distribution of patients according to the presence or absence of a sensory-motor deficit is shown in **Table IV.**

Table IV: Distribution of patients according to sensory-motor deficit.

Number Percentage

Sensory deficit engine	Yes	20	24%
	No	62	76%

With regard to sensory disorders, hypoesthesia was present in all cases. affecting the left L4 root in 02 cases and the L5 and S1 roots in the remaining cases. Only one case of cauda equina syndrome was reported in our series.68 patients had good muscle tone, while the remainder were hypotonic (17%).Pyramidal syndrome was present in only 02 patients in our series.For osteotendinous reflexes, an abnormality of the patellar reflex was noted in 12% of cases and of the achilles reflex in 32% of cases.

I.10 Imaging data :

MRI enabled us to identify :

- Hypertrophy of the yellow ligament in 32 cases.

- Associated narrow cervical canal in 04 cases.

- Zygapophyseal osteoarthritis: 54 cases.

- Signal abnormalities of the discs and vertebral endplates in 68 cases.

- No synovial cysts were detected on any of the MRI images.

- Lumbar muscle degeneration in 36 cases.

- Nerve compression: location and extent.

In our 82 patients, 149 stages were stenotic, as shown in **Table V.**

Table V: Distribution of stenosis according to lumbar level and number of stages.

Stenosis	Number	Percentage
Lumbar level		
L1-L2	01	1%
L2-L3	04	2%
L3-L4	22	15%
L4-L5	64	43%
L5-S1	58	39%
Total	149	100%
Staged stenosis		
1 floor	6	8%
2 floors	41	50%
3 floors	33	40%
4 floors	2	2%

- The degree of stenosis of the rootlets in the dural sac using the Schizas classification. In our series :

Grade A: 49% of cases.

Grade B: 39% of cases.

Grade C: 15% of cases.

Grade D: 2% of cases.

The distribution of patients according to the Schizas classification is shown in the table below. figure 4.

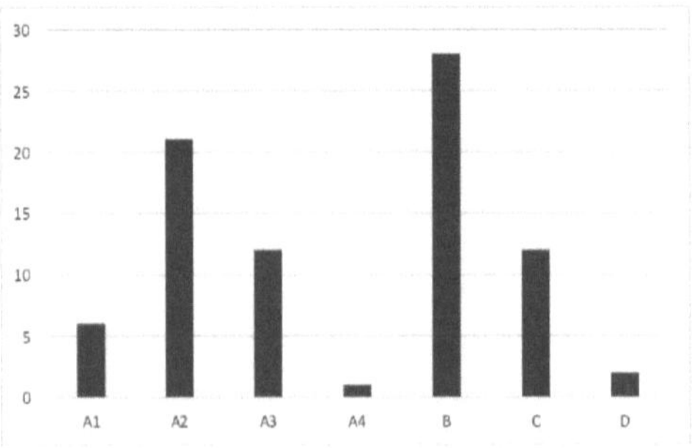

Figure 9: Distribution of patients according to the Schizas classification.

II. CORRELATION OF CLINICAL DATA WITH THE SCHIZAS CLASSIFICATION

The correlation of clinical parameters with the different grades of the Schizas classification is shown in **Table VI**.

Table VI: Correlation of clinical data with the Schizas classification.

	Grade A	Grade B	Grade C	Grade D	P
Perimeter of >500m	16 (40%)	09 (32%)	02 (17%)	0	0,832
walking 100-500m	16 (40%)	08 (29%)	06 (50%)	0	
<100m	08 (20%)	11 (39%)	04 (33%)	02	
Intensity of the Slight	0	0	0	0	0,011
Pain Moderate	15 (38%)	08 (29%)	0	0	
Intense	15 (38%)	08 (29%)	08 (67%)	0	
Unbearable	10 (25%)	12 (42%)	04 (33%)	02	
Reflex Present and patellar symmetrical	36 (90%)	26 (92%)	10 (83%)	0	0,208
Abnormal	04 (10%)	02 (8%)	02 (17%)	02	
Reflex Present and Achilles symmetrical	28 (70%)	26 (81%)	06 (50%)	0	<0,001
Abnormal	12 (30%)	06 (19%)	06 (50%)	02	
Deficit No	36 (90%)	21 (75%)	05 (42%)	0	0,001
sensitivo- Yes engine	04 (10%)	07 (25%)	07 (58%)	02	
Capacity Stage 1	06 (15%)	03 (11%)	0	0	0,089
Functional Stage 2	16 (40%)	10 (36%)	01 (8%)	0	
Stage 3	11 (28%)	10 (36%)	05 (42%)	0	

Stage 4	04 (10%)	05 (17%)	03 (25%)	0	
Stage 5	03 (7%)	0	03 (25%)	02	
Vesico-bladder disorder No	29 (73%)	20 (71%)	08 (67%)	0	0,863
Sphincter Yes	11 (27%)	08 (29%)	04 (33%)	02	

A significant correlation was found between the degree of lumbar stenosis and pain intensity **p=0.011**, the abolition of the achilles reflex **p<0.001** and the sensory-motor deficit **p=0.001**.

We studied 82 patients with a degenerative narrow lumbar canal. We correlated the degree of root stenosis in the dural sac using the Schizas classification to several clinical variables, namely: gait perimeter and neurogenic claudication, pain intensity, functional disability and neurological examination.There was a statistically significant correlation between sensory-motor deficit, pain intensity, abolition of the achilles reflex and Schizas classification. However, our study did not find a statistically significant association between ODI, gait perimeter and neurogenic claudication and Schizas grade.The Schizas classification is a reliable qualitative classification validated by Ko et al.[4] and can be used as a learning method by clinicians and teachers.

radiologists [4].

We consider this work to be original. Several studies have correlated clinical symptoms with quantitative radiological parameters. However, few studies have correlated clinical symptoms with qualitative morphological parameters of the spinal cord using the Schizas classification. This is also the first study in Tunisia to address this subject, according to research on the Tunis Faculty of Medicine website.However, our study had a number of limitations:

- The retrospective, cross-disciplinary nature of the work.

- Limited number of samples.

- Patient records were missing anthropometric data such as weight and height, as well as patients' occupations.

I. DERMOGRAPHIC CHARACTERISTICS

The mean age in our series was 58 years. This average was higher than that found in the literature, such as in the series by Jain [37], whereas it was lower than that in the series by Weber [35], Aaen [38], Andrasinova [34] and Moojen [39].

In the literature, men are more often affected by degenerative changes of the lumbar spine than women [40]. Unlike the series by Jain [37], Weber [35], Aaen [38], Moojen [39] and Andrasinova [34], our series was predominantly female. **Table VII** summarises the mean ages and gender proportions reported in the literature.

Table VII: Average age and gender of patients with a root canal degenerative narrow lumbar spine in the literature.

	Year	Proportion of men (%)	Average ages (years)
Aaen	2022	52,7	66,8
Jain	2020		53,67
Moojen	2018	53	66
Andrasinova	2018	50	70
Weber	2016	55 ,5	68,1
Our series	2022	43	58

Canal stenosis becomes symptomatic from the 5^e decade [41] because ageing leads to degeneration and changes in the anatomy of the lumbar spine [3,4]. Anatomically [3], central canal stenosis may result from a decrease in anteroposterior, transverse or combined diameter, secondary to loss of disc height with or without bulging of the intervertebral disc, and hypertrophy of the facet joints and yellow ligament due to fibrosis. Lateral stenosis may result from posterolateral osteophytes of the vertebral plates protruding into the foramen, as well as annular fibrosis or a laterally bulging disc herniation which compresses the nerve root against the superior pedicle.

II. STUDIES OF DATA FROM THE INTERVIEW AND PHYSICAL EXAMINATION

II. 1. Walking distance and neurogenic claudication :

We found no significant correlation between gait circumference and Schizas grades. Jain [37], Weber [35], Aaen [38], Moojen [39] and Andrasinova [34] concurred with this finding and confirmed the absence of a link between gait circumference and Schizas classification.

II. 2. Pain intensity :

Our study found a correlation between VAS and the degree of stenosis on MRI. However, the literature contradicts our results [34,35,37-39] . The discrepancy between our results and those of the literature could be explained by the predominance of women in our series, in contrast to series in the literature. Indeed, Yeom [42] has shown that women present with greater lumbar pain and low back pain than men. This difference in symptom severity may be partially mediated by pain sensitivity.

II. 3. Functional disability :

We found no correlation between ODI and the degree of lumbar canal stenosis. Our results are in line with those of Jain [37], Weber [35], Aaen [38], Moojen [39] and Andrasinova [34].There may be several reasons for the poor correlation between radiological findings and clinical symptoms, as a narrow canal is only one factor in the pathogenesis of neurogenic claudication [34]. Kuittinen [14] argued that the narrow lumbar canal is not just an anatomical disorder but that the disease may have other underlying pathobiological mechanisms. He stressed that adaptive mechanisms have a role to play in that pain can disappear spontaneously over time and longer walking distances become feasible. Kuittinen [14] and Genevay [1] concluded that intermittent hypoxia of the ponytail roots resulting from venous congestion and failure of arterial vasodilatation of the congested roots has been proposed as a physio-pathological mechanism underlying neurogenic claudication. Furthermore, the lack of a clear relationship between imaging findings and the clinical presentation of stenosis could be explained by the fact that conventional MRI is performed in the supine position, whereas symptoms of stenosis are generally precipitated by standing or walking. In the upright position, the spinal canal may be narrowed by segmental instability, compression by soft tissue structures (synovial cyst, yellow ligament, intervertebral disc, posterior epidural fat) or venous congestion [16].Kanno [43] and Zhou [44] have shown that the size of the dural sac on loaded axial MRI was reduced and significantly correlated with the severity of symptoms.

II. 4. Sensory-motor deficit :

We found a significant correlation between sensory-motor deficit and Schizas classification. This is in line with the study by Andrasinova [34], who found a tendency for a more pronounced neurological deficit in the lower limbs of patients with more severe central stenosis (Schizas grade D classification).

III. INTEREST OF THE QUALITATIVE EVALUATION OF THE LUMBAR CANAL IN MRI AND THE THERAPEUTIC IMPACT

In the literature, the majority of studies have correlated the size and measurements of the lumbar canal with the clinical situation. Amudsen et al [10] found no relationship between the degree of stenosis (measured by myelography and CT scan) and clinical symptoms in 100 patients selected from a neurology centre on the basis of clinical symptoms of CLE.Lohman et al [11] found no relationship between canal cross-sectional area measured by CT scan and clinical symptoms.Sirvanci et al [12] studied the correlation between imaging and ODI in 63 surgical candidates with CLE. They studied cross-sectional area, but found no correlation between these parameters and ODI. Jonsson et al [13] observed a non-significant trend towards gait disturbance in patients with CLE with more pronounced stenosis observed on myelography. Kuittinen et al [14] and Zeifang et al [15] showed that there was no association between lumbar canal stenosis and functional capacity based on MRI measurement of dural sac surface area.Haig et al [16] pointed out that MRI had no discriminatory value in distinguishing between patients with severe clinical stenosis of asymptomatic volunteers. None of the studies mentioned above looked at qualitative morphological characteristics and were limited to trying to establish a relationship between the parameters measured and symptoms or functional status. Nevertheless, assessment of CLE using a grading system was widely used in clinical practice. Schizas et al [8] suggested a 4-grade classification based on dural sac morphology with consideration of the root canal to cerebrospinal fluid (CSF) ratio on MRI. Due to its ability to perform a rapid visual assessment without the need for specific measuring tools, the MRI qualitative classification system has been widely used in clinical reports as radiological parameters to classify CLE.The diagnosis of neurogenic claudication is an important clinical decision because it determines the therapeutic management. The presence of ductal narrowing is only a secondary confirmatory element. The fact that radiological findings are not associated with clinical symptoms confirms the general conclusion that lumbar canal narrowing is very often asymptomatic. Indeed, Tong et al [17] studied central lumbar canal stenosis in asymptomatic patients over 55 years of age; 72.8% had at least mild central stenosis, 30.3% had at least moderate stenosis, and 6.1% had severe stenosis present in at least one level. According to our study, it is not possible to estimate clinical symptoms or the degree of disability in patients with CLE on the basis of MRI findings. We agree with the idea that CLE is a clinico-radiological syndrome with complex relationship between the degree of radiological stenosis and clinical manifestations. Radiological findings alone are insufficient to justify treatment of canal stenosis, and for good reason. MRI is performed in the supine position, which cancels out the dynamic compression effect of the mobile spinal segment. The choice of treatment (surgery or conservative treatment) for patients with CLE should be based on the degree of clinical involvement.

CONCLUSION

Degenerative narrow lumbar canal is a frequent pathology from the fifth decade onwards. It corresponds to a maladjustment of the lumbar spine's container-content ratio.

Clinically, the main symptom is intermittent neurogenic claudication. Cauda equina syndrome is a serious condition, but it is rare and seems to be linked to a progressive stage of the disease.

Degenerative lumbar spinal stenosis is diagnosed clinically and radiologically. As MRI is the gold standard for diagnosing LRS, several MRI-based classification systems have been proposed to assess the severity of this disorder. However, the patient's perception of the symptoms is not always compatible with the radiological findings, and this is the subject of debate. CLE is an anatomo-clinical syndrome with complex relationships between the degree of stenosis and clinical manifestations. The literature contains studies that describe a weak relationship between the size of the lumbar canal and clinical symptoms.

Our study is a retrospective, descriptive study of 82 patients followed for degenerative narrow lumbar canal. It was based on the Schizas classification, which is a qualitative morphological classification. It describes the morphology of the dural sac, observed on T2 axial magnetic resonance images, as a function of the radicle/cerebrospinal fluid ratio.

We were interested in correlating clinical symptoms with the degree of root stenosis in the dural sac, assessed by the Schizas classification on MRI.

Our study found a significant correlation between the grade of stenosis of the cauda equina rootlets and motor deficit (p=0.001) and pain intensity (p=0.011). However, we did not identify any association between the degree of stenosis and functional disability (ODI) or walking capacity (gait perimeter).

In fact, absolute estimation of clinical symptoms or degree of disability in patients with CLE was not possible on the basis of MRI findings. Radiological findings alone are insufficient to define the severity of the pathology and to justify treatment of ductal stenosis. Therefore, the choice of treatment (surgery or conservative treatment) in patients with CLE should be based on the degree of clinical involvement.

REFERENCES

[1] Genevay S, Chevallier-Ruggeri P, Faundez A. [Lumbar spinal stenosis: clinical course, pathophysiology and treatment]. Rev Med Suisse. 14 March 2012;8(332):585-6, 588-9.

[2] Lafian AM, Torralba KD. Lumbar Spinal Stenosis in Older Adults. Rheum Dis Clin North Am. August 2018;44(3):501-12.

[3] Genevay S, Atlas SJ. Lumbar spinal stenosis. Best Pract Res Clin Rheumatol. Apr 2010;24(2):253-65.

[4] Ko Y jee, Lee E, Lee JW, Park CY, Cho J, Kang Y, et al. Clinical validity of two different grading systems for lumbar central canal stenosis: Schizas and Lee classification systems. PLoS One. 27 May 2020;15(5):e0233633.

[5] Park S, Han HS, Kim GU, Kang SS, Kim HJ, Lee M, et al. Relationships among Disability, Quality of Life, and Physical Fitness in Lumbar Spinal Stenosis: An Investigation of Elderly Korean Women. Asian Spine J. Apr 2017;11(2):256-63.

[6] Özdemir E, Paker N, Bugdayci D, Tekdos DD. Quality of life and related factors in degenerative lumbar spinal stenosis: A controlled study. J Back Musculoskelet Rehabil. 2015;28(4):749-53.

[7] Olmarker K, Rydevik B, Hansson T, Holm S. Compression-induced changes of the nutritional supply to the porcine cauda equina. J Spinal Disord. March 1990;3(1):25-9.

[8] Schizas C, Theumann N, Burn A, Tansey R, Wardlaw D, Smith FW, et al. Qualitative grading of severity of lumbar spinal stenosis based on the morphology of the dural sac on magnetic resonance images. Spine (Phila Pa 1976). 1 Oct 2010;35(21):1919-24.

[9] Lim YS, Mun JU, Seo MS, Sang BH, Bang YS, Kang KN, et al.

Dural sac area is a more sensitive parameter for evaluating lumbar spinal stenosis than spinal canal area: A retrospective study. Medicine (Baltimore). dec 2017;96(49):e9087.

[10]Amundsen T, Weber H, Lilleås F, Nordal HJ, Abdelnoor M, Magnaes B. Lumbar spinal stenosis. Clinical and radiologic features. Spine (Phila Pa 1976). 15 May 1995;20(10):1178-86.

[11]Lohman CM, Tallroth K, Kettunen JA, Lindgren KA. Comparison of radiologic signs and clinical symptoms of spinal stenosis. Spine (Phila Pa 1976). 15 Jul 2006;31(16):1834-40.

[12] Sirvanci M, Bhatia M, Ganiyusufoglu KA, Duran C, Tezer M, Ozturk C, et al. Degenerative lumbar spinal stenosis: correlation with Oswestry Disability Index and MR Imaging. Eur Spine J. May 2008;17(5):679-85.

[13] Jönsson B, Annertz M, Sjöberg C, Strömqvist B. A prospective and consecutive study of surgically treated lumbar spinal stenosis. Part I: Clinical features related to radiographic findings. Spine (Phila Pa 1976). 15 Dec 1997;22(24):2932-7.

[14] Kuittinen P, Sipola P, Saari T, Aalto TJ, Sinikallio S, Savolainen S, et al. Visually assessed severity of lumbar spinal canal stenosis is paradoxically associated with leg pain and objective walking ability. BMC Musculoskeletal Disord. 16 Oct 2014;15:348.

[15] Zeifang F, Schiltenwolf M, Abel R, Moradi B. Gait analysis does not correlate with clinical and MR imaging parameters in patients with symptomatic lumbar spinal stenosis. BMC Musculoskeletal Disord. 20 June 2008;9:89.

[16] Haig AJ, Tomkins CC. Diagnosis and management of lumbar spinal stenosis. JAMA. 6 Jan 2010;303(1):71-2.

[17] Tong HC, Carson JT, Haig AJ, Quint DJ, Phalke VR, Yamakawa KSJ, et al. Magnetic resonance imaging of the lumbar spine in asymptomatic older adults. Journal of Back and Musculoskeletal Rehabilitation. 1 Jan 2006;19(2-3):67-72.

[18] Kim YU, Kong YG, Lee J, Cheong Y, Kim S hun, Kim HK, et al. Clinical symptoms of lumbar spinal stenosis associated with morphological parameters on magnetic resonance images. Eur Spine J. Oct 2015;24(10):2236-43.

[19] Arabmotlagh M, Sellei RM, Vinas-Rios JM, Rauschmann M. [Classification and diagnosis of lumbar spinal stenosis]. Orthopade. oct 2019;48(10):816-23.

[20] Burgstaller JM, Schüffler PJ, Buhmann JM, Andreisek G, Winklhofer S, Del Grande F, et al. Is There an Association Between Pain and Magnetic Resonance Imaging Parameters in Patients With Lumbar Spinal Stenosis? Spine (Phila Pa 1976). Sep 2016;41(17):E1053-62.

[21] Huang CC, Jaw FS, Young YH. Radiological and functional assessment in patients with lumbar spinal stenosis. BMC Musculoskeletal Disord. Feb 10, 2022;23(1):137.

[22] Schizas C, Kulik G. Decision-making in lumbar spinal stenosis. The Journal of Bone and Joint Surgery British volume. Jan 2012;94-B(1):98-101.

[23] Fairbank JC, Pynsent PB. The Oswestry Disability Index. Spine (Phila Pa 1976). 15 Nov 2000;25(22):2940-52; discussion 2952.

[24] Huskisson EC. Measurement of pain. Lancet. 9 Nov 1974;2(7889):1127-31.

[25]Bodian CA, Freedman G, Hossain S, Eisenkraft JB, Beilin Y. The

Visual Analog Scale for Pain: Clinical Significance in Postoperative Patients. Anesthesiology. Dec 1, 2001;95(6):1356-61.

[26]Skovlund E, Breivik H. Analysis of pain-intensity measurements. Scand J Pain. Oct 2016;13:123-4.

[27]Deer T, Sayed D, Michels J, Josephson Y, Li S, Calodney AK. A Review of Lumbar Spinal Stenosis with Intermittent Neurogenic Claudication: Disease and Diagnosis. Pain Med. Dec 2019;20(Suppl 2):S32-44.

[28]Robert K. Snider. Essentials of Musculoskeletal Care [Internet]. Rosemont, Illinois, U.S.a.: Amer Academy of Orthopaedic; 2001 [cited 19 Jul 2022]. Available from: https://www.biblio.com/book/essentials-musculoskeletal-care-robert-k-snider/d/1457596024

[29] Murtagh J. Schober's test (modified). Aust Fam Physician. July 1989;18(7):849.

[30]Cidem M, Karacan I, Uludag M. Normal range of spinal mobility for healthy young adult Turkish men. Rheumatol Int. August 2012;32(8):2265-9.

[31]M Das J, Nadi M. Lasegue Sign. In: StatPearls [Internet]. Treasure Island (FL): StatPearls Publishing; 2022 [cited 16 Jul 2022]. Available from: http://www.ncbi.nlm.nih.gov/books/NBK545299/

[32]Hislop HJ, Avers D, Brown M, editors. Chapter 1 - Principles of manual muscle testing. In: Daniels and Worthingham muscle testing (9th edition) [Internet]. Paris: Elsevier Masson; 2015 [cited 16 Jul 2022]. p. 1-9. Available from: https://www.sciencedirect.com/science/article/pii/B9782294739941000010

[33]Maintaining the capacities of myopaths or the art of prescribing physical exercise [Internet]. RevueMedicale Switzerland. [cited 19 July 2022]. Available from at: https://www.revmed.ch/revue-medicale-suisse/2014/revue-medicale-suisse- 428/maintien-des-capacites-des-myopathes-ou-l'-art-de-prescrire-l-exercice-physique

[34]Andrasinova T, Adamova B, Buskova J, Kerkovsky M, Jarkovsky J, Bednarik J. Is there a Correlation Between Degree of Radiologic Lumbar Spinal Stenosis and its Clinical Manifestation? Clinical Spine Surgery: A Spine Publication. Oct 2018;31(8):E403-8.

[35] Weber C, Giannadakis C, Rao V, Jakola AS, Nerland U, Nygaard ØP, et al. Is There an Association Between Radiological Severity of Lumbar Spinal Stenosis and Disability, Pain, or Surgical Outcome: A Multicenter Observational Study. SPINE. Jan 2016;41(2):E78-83.

[36] P. Vandermarcq, S. Velasco, P. Ardilouze, S. Boucebci. Stenosis of the lumbar canal [Internet]. EM-Consulte. 2011 [cited 16 Jul 2022]. Available from: https://www.em-consulte.com/article/286735/stenoses-du-canal-lombaire

[37] Jain N, Acharya S, Adsul NM, Haritwal MK, Kumar M, Chahal RS, et al. Lumbar Canal Stenosis: A Prospective Clinicoradiologic Analysis. J Neurol Surg A Cent Eur Neurosurg. Sept 2020;81(5):387-91.

[38] Aaen J, Austevoll IM, Hellum C, Storheim K, Myklebust TÅ, Banitalebi H, et al. Clinical and MRI findings in lumbar spinal stenosis: baseline data from the NORDSTEN study. Eur Spine J. 1 June 2022;31(6):1391-8.

[39] Moojen WA, Schenck CD, Lycklama À Nijeholt GJ, Jacobs WCH, Van der Kallen BF, Arts MP, et al. Preoperative MRI in

Patients With Intermittent Neurogenic Claudication: Relevance for Diagnosis and Prognosis. Spine (Phila Pa 1976). March 1, 2018;43(5):348-55.

[40] Suthar P, Patel R, Mehta C, Patel N. MRI Evaluation of Lumbar Disc Degenerative Disease. J Clin Diagn Res. Apr 2015;9(4):TC04-9.

[41] Sheehan JM, Shaffrey CI, Jane JA. Degenerative lumbar stenosis: the neurosurgical perspective. Clin Orthop Relat Res. March 2001;(384):61-74.

[42] Yeom JS. Gender Difference of Symptom Severity inLumbar Spinal Stenosis: Role of Pain Sensitivity. Pain Phys. Nov 14, 2013;6;16(6;11):E715-23.

[43] Kanno H, Ozawa H, Koizumi Y, Morozumi N, Aizawa T, Kusakabe T, et al. Dynamic change of dural sac cross-sectional area in axial loaded magnetic resonance imaging correlates with the severity of clinical symptoms in patients with lumbar spinal canal stenosis. Spine (Phila Pa 1976). Feb 1, 2012;37(3):207-13.

[44] Zhou Z, Jin Z, Zhang P, Shan B, Zhou Z, Zhang Y, et al. Correlation Between Dural Sac Size in Dynamic Magnetic Resonance Imaging and Clinical Symptoms in Patients with Lumbar Spinal Stenosis. World Neurosurgery. 1 Feb 2020;134:e866-73.

APPENDIXES

Appendix 1: Operating sheet

Surname/First name :

Genre :

Age :

Reason for consultation: Previous

history :

Medical :

Surgical :

 Profession :

Development time :

Functional signs :

• Chronic low back pain :

• Lower back pain:

o Head office:

o Type :

• Type of pain :

• Intermittent medullary claudication :

 • walking perimeter :

• Genito-sphincter disorders:

• EVA :

• ODI :

• Cervicobrachial neuralgia:

 Physical signs :

• walk: Talon :

       Toes :

• Examination of the spine :

o Lumbar stiffness :

o Analgesic attitude :

o Sign of the bell :

o Lasègue sign :

o Neurological examination :

o Motor disorders

o Sensory disorders :

o Ponytail syndrome :

o muscle tone :

o ROT [Achillean/Rotulian] :

o pyramidal syndrome :

Radiological examination :

• MRI :

CLE :

    -   -disco-radicular conflict

    -   -Zygapophyseal osteoarthritis

    -   -Synovial cyst

    -   -hypertrophy of the yellow ligament

    -   -number of floors :

    -   -muscle degeneration :

    -   -Schizas classification :

Treatment :

• Medical :

• Rehabilitation :

Evolution :

Appendix 2: Oswestry disability index

Section 1: Pain Intensity

0. [illegible]
1. [illegible]
2. [illegible]
3. [illegible]
4. [illegible]
5. [illegible]

Section 2: Personal Care

0. [illegible]
1. [illegible]
2. [illegible]
3. [illegible]
4. [illegible]
5. [illegible]

Section 3: Lifting

0. [illegible]
1. [illegible]
2. [illegible]
3. [illegible]
4. [illegible]
5. [illegible]

Section 4: Walking

0. [illegible]
1. [illegible]
2. [illegible]
3. [illegible]
4. [illegible]
5. [illegible]

Section 5: Sitting

0. [illegible]
1. [illegible]
2. [illegible]
3. [illegible]
4. [illegible]
5. [illegible]

Section 6: Standing

0. [illegible]
1. [illegible]
2. [illegible]
3. [illegible]
4. [illegible]
5. [illegible]

Section 7: Sleeping

0. [illegible]
1. [illegible]
2. [illegible]
3. [illegible]
4. [illegible]

Section 8: Social Life

0. [illegible]
1. [illegible]
2. [illegible]
3. [illegible]
4. [illegible]
5. [illegible]

Section 9: Traveling

0. [illegible]
1. [illegible]
2. [illegible]
3. [illegible]
4. [illegible]
5. [illegible]

Section 10: Changing Degree of Pain

0. [illegible]
1. [illegible]
2. [illegible]
3. [illegible]
4. [illegible]
5. [illegible]

Oswestry disability index [23].

Appendix 3: Visual analogue scale

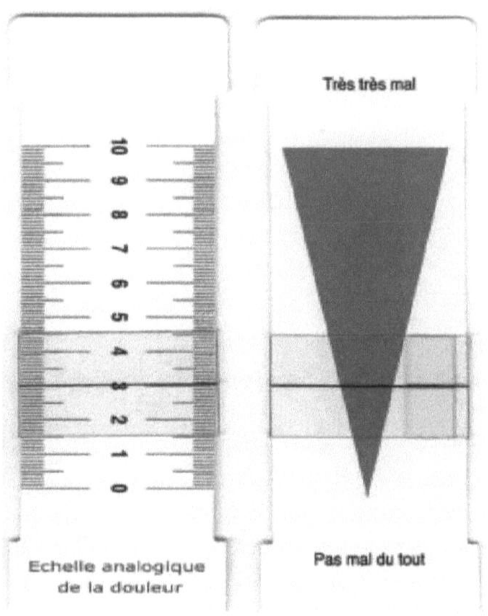

Diagram of the visual analogue scale [25].

Appendix 4: Comparison of neurogenic claudication and vascular claudication

	Vascular claudication	Neurogenic claudication
Walking distance	Fixed	Variable
Pain relief	Stand up	Sitting and/or leaning forward
Walking uphill	Limb pain lower	No pain
Cycling	Limb pain lower	No pain
Type of pain	Cramping, tightening	Numbness, stinging
Foot pulse	Absent	Normal
Skin on limbs lower	Hair loss and atrophy	Normal
Muscular atrophy of the legs	Rare	Occasional
Weak limbs lower	Rare	Occasional
Back pain	Not usual	Usual
Limited mobility spinal	Not usual	Usual

Comparison of neurogenic and vascular claudication [28].

Appendix 5: Scoring muscle strength

46

0 = Aucune contraction
1 = Contraction visible n'entraînant aucun mouvement
2 = Contraction permettant le mouvement en l'absence de pesanteur
3 = Contraction permettant le mouvement contre la pesanteur
4 = Contraction permettant le mouvement contre la résistance
5 = Force musculaire normale

Muscle strength scoring table [32,33].

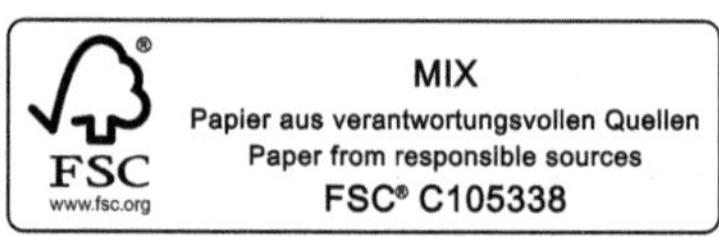

Printed by Books on Demand GmbH, Norderstedt / Germany